Terms and Conditions

LEGAL NOTICE

Table Of Contents

Foreword

Chapter1:
Introduction To Your New Life

Chapter2:
Basics To Breaking Old Habits

Chapter 3:
Nutritional Tips For Conquering Ciggy Cravings

Chapter 4:
Benefits of Meditation

Chapter 5:
Affirmations for Abstinence

Chapter 6:
Healthy Habits For A Better Life

Wrapping Up

Foreword

Are you a nicotine addict? The unmatched property that displays the addictive nature of nicotine isn't how hard or how simple it is to stop, nor is it how hard or easy it is for a person to stay off nicotine. The one true property that presents the might of the addiction is that irrespective how long a person is off, one puff and that declaration to stop can go out the window.

Don't ever try to tell yourself that you weren't addicted. You were addicted to nicotine all of the years you utilized it and you're addicted to it now too. However as an ex-smoker the addiction becomes asymptomatic. To keep it that way and to always stay in command, remember to never pick up another smoke! Get all the info you need here.

Cigarette Crusher
Easy Ways To Eliminate Smoking Addiction And Revitalize Your Body

Chapter 1:

Introduction To Your New Life

Synopsis

I know that if you are a smoker it may be difficult to quit. However, if you wish to stop you will. You'll get the willpower to take charge. Smoking isn't good for anybody. Second hand, smoke has proven to be worse than smoking. For those around you, once you smoke you're hurting them too. Many individuals smoke for years, which make it hard to quit. Nevertheless, you have help and hope, particularly if you wish to quit bad enough.

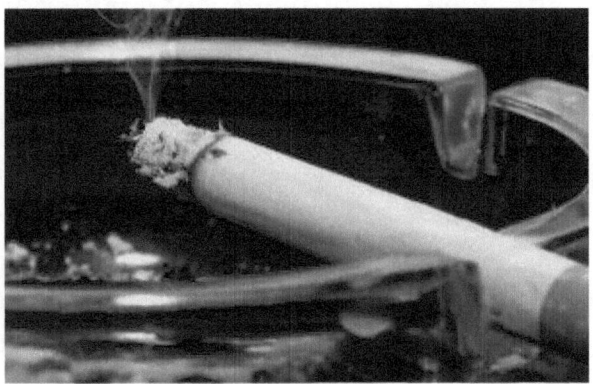

The Basics

Preventing unhealthy living:

Why do individuals begin smoking? A few individuals begin smoking because they think it's something cool and their friends are impressed. They believe it makes them look mature. Regrettably, many individuals begin smoking early in life. Many individuals regrettably end up with bronchitis, breathing issues, cancer, and lung disease and so on. As teenagers, we thought it was the cool thing to do, as all of our friends were doing it. We might have picked up the habit watching parents or grandparents smoke.

How smoking impacts you:

No one knows what would happen to you if you don't quit until the time comes for you to know. You may get cancer in your mouth, in your lungs, you might have a difficult time breathing, fast heartbeat, you might have problems walking across the room. Many things might happen to you if you don't quit. Ironically, however, a few individuals smoke for years and nothing happens to them. Yet, throughout the years these individuals feel sluggish, tired, and frequently get colds more often.

The advantages of stopping smoking:

Just think if you quit smoking you won't have to worry about the smell in your home, in your car or on your clothes. You won't have those nasty ash trays to empty or wash. You won't have to smell nothing but the air you breathe. If you quit now you'll begin to get

back yourself. You'll be able to walk across the floor or be able to breathe without using oxygen to help you there are a lot of reasons to quit, I wish you the best.

A few of the reasons individuals don't quit smoking are because they believe they'll gain weight.

Contrary to your notions, smoking will make you gain weight as you begin to age. To improve personal life you must take measures to protect your overall health, which includes maintaining weight, quit smoking and so on. The steps you take will lead you to a healthier future and a successful conclusion.

If you're finding it hard to beat the habit, we encourage you to learn about the drugs inside cigarettes. If it isn't enough to scare you into stopping now, then consider your future, living on life-support or oxygen tanks.

Chapter 2:

Basics To Breaking Old Habits

Synopsis

Change is all about results. If you remain off cigarettes and you're living a satisfying life then that's good. You've exposed your calling and whatever plan (or lack thereof) that you're working appears to be the right fit for you.

In other words, if you're attempting to recover from an addiction, the best thing to do is to do what figures out for you. Instead of taking a hard-line on precisely what needs to be achieved in order to recover, traditional wisdom states you should explore and find what works best.

Where To Start

If someone acquaints you with a program--any plan at all--you must be realistic about it. Recognize that any plan for change is truly just a collection of suggestions. If a change plan is going to work for you, do you think it's the actual suggestions of the program that bring about the results, or do you think that the results bank more heavily on your personal actions? Just how complicated is a plan of change, truly? It's not what you do; it's how you achieve it. Consider what a great change plan truly consists of. We might break it down like this:

1) Abstinence

2) A blueprint for living

3) Support and networking (assisting others)

4) Personal maturation

Really, where is the mystery in this? Certainly, it's a lot of stuff. And no, it's not unavoidably simple to achieve. Individuals fail at change again and again. But my point is that there's no grand mystery in the plan itself. The answers are in the action.

There's a shift that occurs once the struggling addict in early on change is no more battling to remain free of nicotine; they discover a particular peace about themselves and things start clicking for them. Either that or they relapse. However the idea of transition is real.

Change is split into short-term and long-run change. We do particular things to begin with to remain clean. If we don't alter our strategy eventually and make the transition to long-run change, we relapse. We must change in order to make it over the long run.

We must achieve particular things in early on change to remain clean. These are different things for everyone, but the precepts are the same: we require a strong support system, much structure; some require protection from the outside world (like a treatment center). Still these things won't keep you clean 5 years down the road or even one year out. Those who don't changeover to long-run, holistic living will inevitably slide back into their old behaviors.

No one consciously knows once they're making this jump from short-term to long-run change. It simply occurs. You're able to retrospect, naturally, and discover how you grew through the stage.

So how may we know what to do? How may we help the changeover? The answer to this is what the originative theory is all about. The answer lies in the 3 primary techniques:

1) Treasuring self

2) Networking with others

3) Push for holistic maturation

Particularly, the push for holistic maturation is a critical component of the transition. I'm not so certain that you're able to plan this sort of growth out specifically, however. What's crucial is to get past the mentality of "I'm just going to focus on my plan and not get distracted with schooling or career or additional things right now." Many traditional plans don't encourage holistic maturation so if you focus on them then you're going to be doing so at the exclusion of additional growth opportunities.

All the same maturation involves change. We either move onward in change or we slide back.

So my proposal is to seek holistic growth opportunities right from the beginning. Find ways to diversify and grow or learn outside of the limits of "traditional change." This may include things like physical fitness, nutrition, meditation, training, the arts, learning new skills, building new relationships, etcetera.

The transition occurs once you grow beyond the minute focus of your early change efforts. Once we're working a traditional plan of change, we tend to have a restricted view in that we perceive all potential growth as being one-dimensional. Maybe the twelve step model has facilitated this idea as the twelve steps are plainly ordered and are in sequence.

Still in holistic living, maturation may be expansive and non-linear. Regardless what program you're working, most individuals don't grow at a regular pace in change. Many of us careen around for a while to begin with, trying to find our footing and merely get through the cravings and urges of every day. Later on, once we have been making holistic growth attempts, our maturation in change may be explosive.

In other words, at times we have to slog through a tough time in change once we see little results from our attempts. The payoff comes eventually once all of our holistic maturation attempts begin paying off down the road at some point.

The only real enemy in long-run change is complacency. After living nicotine free, we no longer battle with daily urges or even with more elusive threats to change like resentments or self-pity. Rather, the true challenge in long-term change is to continue challenging ourselves to mature.

Center on the 3 primary techniques and continue pushing yourself to grow, and complacency will take care of itself. Once we're first beginning in change, there are a few high impact matters that we may do in order to get going on the right foot. These are action oriented matters we may do, like:

1) Attend treatment

2) Attend meetings

3) Call our sponsor or additional recovering addicts

4) Examine change literature or write up step work

And so forth. These are the sorts of things that are normally suggested to newbies in change. Why? Because they work. They help.

Best is to challenge yourself to mature in your change and develop as a spiritual being. What does this entail? It means that instead of ditching your issues and sniveling in a meeting daily, you ought to be spending your energy in richer ways as you advance in change. One way to achieve this would be to provide addiction help to others.

You may likewise seek to discover new ways to grow outside of the limits of traditional change. For example, the twelve step plan typically centers on spiritual growth solely. This is a shortsighted viewpoint and to really recover you have to heal your life in additional ways too, including physically, emotionally, socially, etc. In order to recover, you have to live this way.

Chapter 3:

Nutritional Tips For Conquering Ciggy Cravings

Synopsis

Blood sugar plummets in a lot of People when first quitting. The commonest side effects experienced during the first days might frequently be traced back to blood sugar issues. Symptoms like headache, inability to focus, vertigo, time sensing distortions, and the ubiquitous sweet tooth found by many, are frequently affiliated with this blood sugar drop.

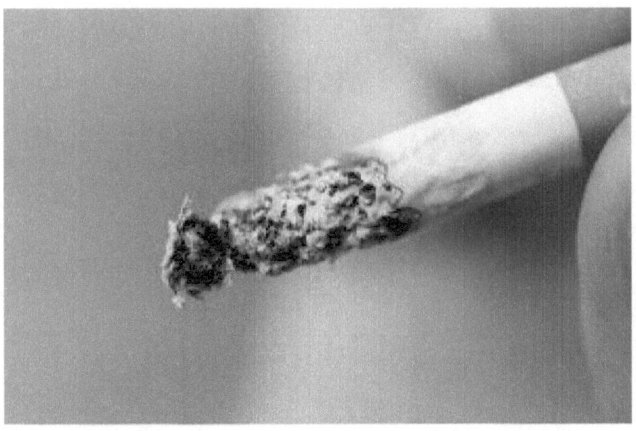

Think About The Food

The symptoms of low blood sugar are essentially the same symptoms as not getting enough oxygen, similar to reactions experienced at high altitudes. The reason being the poor supply of sugar and/or oxygen means the brain is getting an incomplete fuel. If you've plenty of one and not plenty of the other, your brain can't operate at any sort of optimal level. Once you quit smoking, oxygen levels are frequently better than they've been in a while, however with a modified supply of sugar it can't properly fuel your brain.

If you use food to raise blood sugar levels, it literally takes up to 20 minutes from the time you chew and swallow the food before it's discharged to the blood, and thus the brain, for its desired effect of fueling your brain. Cigarettes, by carrying out a drug interaction get the body to give up its own stores of sugar, however not in twenty minutes however commonly in a matter of minutes. In a way, your body hasn't had to give up sugar from food in years; you've done it by utilizing nicotine's drug effect!

This is why many People truly gorge themselves on food upon quitting. They start to go through a drop in blood sugar and instinctively get hold of something sweet. Upon finishing the food, they still feel symptoms. Naturally they do, it takes them a moment or two to eat, however the blood sugar isn't hiked up for another 18 minutes. As they're not feeling instantly better, they devour a bit

more. They carry on eating increasingly more food, moment after moment till they at last start to feel better.

Again if they're waiting for the blood glucose to go up we're talking of 20 minutes after the 1ST swallow. People may eat a lot of food in 20 minutes. However they start to trust that this was the amount required before feeling better. This may be replicated many times throughout the day therefore causing many calories being ingested and inducing weight gain to become a real risk.

Once you abruptly quit smoking, the body is in sort of a state of loss, not willful how to work normally as it hasn't worked normally in such a while. Generally by the 3rd day, however, your body will readjust and relinquish sugar as it's required. Without consuming any more your body will simply work out how to govern blood sugar more efficiently.

You may find however that you do have to change dietary patterns to one that's more regular for you. Regular isn't what it was as a smoker, however more what it was before you took up smoking . A few People go till evening without eating while they're smokers. If they attempt the same process as ex-smokers they'll have side effects of low blood sugar.

It isn't that there's something wrong with them now; they were abnormal previously for all pragmatic purposes. This doesn't mean they should consume more food, however it may mean they have to

redistribute the food consumed to a more scattered pattern so they're getting blood sugar doses throughout the day as nature truly had always intended.

To downplay a few of the true low blood sugar effects of the first few days it truly might help to drink juice throughout the day. After the 4th day however, this should no longer be essential as your body should be able to give up sugar stores if your diet is normalized.

If you're having problems that are indicative of blood sugar issues beyond day 3, it wouldn't hurt speaking to your doctor and perchance acquiring some nutritionary counseling.

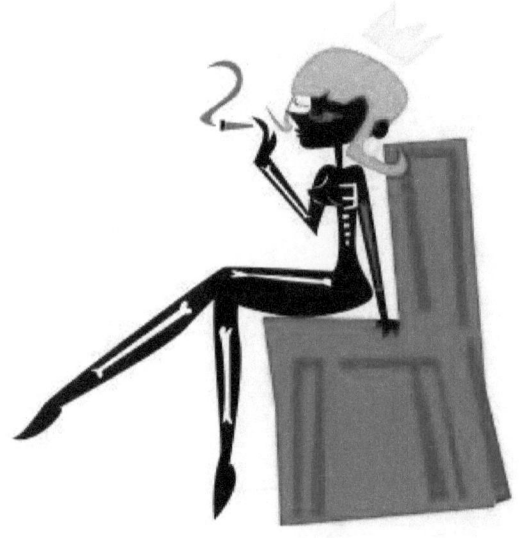

Chapter 4:

Benefits of Meditation

Synopsis

Decently executed meditative breathing sessions may contribute to the arresting of treating of respiratory sickness. In a few severe cases the aid of a breathing apparatus is paramount in ensuring the person gets the vital air needed to continue functioning. Utilizing meditative breathing techniques it's possible to slowly wean these patients of the breathing machine.

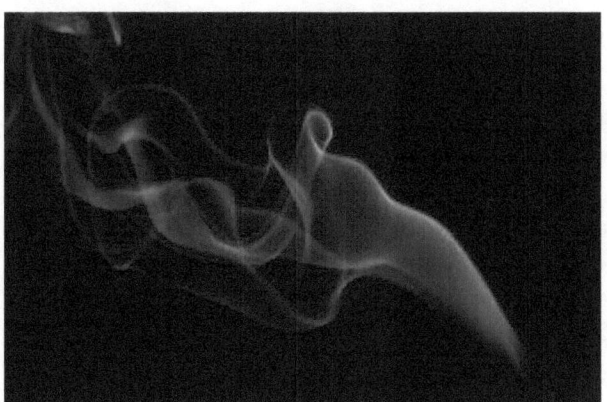

Calming

As the first and commonest steps in meditation sessions call for the practice of breathing, and becoming very aware of the sounds and feelings this breathing makes, the person is able to train the brain to adjust this breathing patters to suit the need at hand.

Like any other muscles in the body, the diaphragm may get "slothful" when not used to its optimal workings, so through meditation the person is encouraged to visualize the actual diaphragm enlarging, and contracting until the desired optimal state is attained.

These deep breathing exercises are only good if the meditation session is done consistently and cautiously. The deep even slow movements of breathing caused by meditation calms the mind and body.

Through meditative breathing methods, the breath in the lung cavity is increased and this helps to increase the oxygen levels in the blood stream, which successively harmonizes the mind and body to combat any respiratory sickness effectively.

Many respiratory diseases obstruct the breathing patterns at assorted stages, due to blockages. Simply breathing harder or faster won't help the congestion. All the same the meditative style of breathing exercises produces better and fuller breaths.

A few illnesses require particular styles of meditative breathing. Asthma is one select example. Although asthma manifests as a physical symptom, a healthy breathing strategy will help the person address the emotional state of mind that bring on such an attack.

Bronchial asthma is a different respiratory sickness that may be helped by meditative breathing exercises. Perhaps not to the extent of curing the disease but surely to help make the patient more comfortable and less stressed.

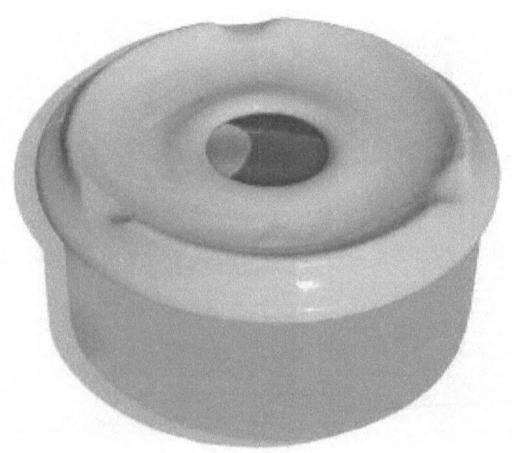

Chapter 5:

Affirmations for Abstinence

Synopsis

You are able to utilize affirmations to get yourself thinking and feeling that you do not wish to smoke. All the same, you do not wish to put in references to smoking in your affirmations, merely as you already have a notion that smoking is enjoyable. Once that association has been made in your subconscious mind, any idea of smoking is going to activate a potent desire to smoke.

Rather, you are able to use affirmations to emphasize the benefits of not smoking - without bringing up smoking at all.

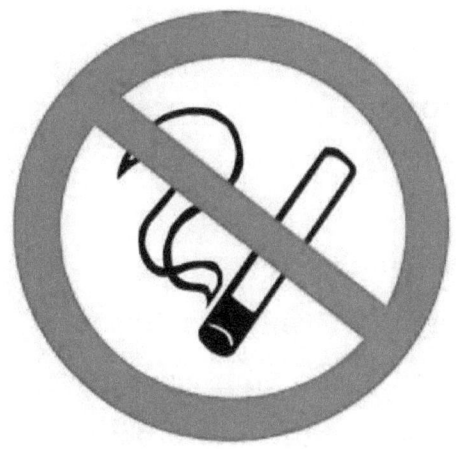

Affirming It

Here are a few examples:

- I love being able to breathe freely.

- I love taking exceptional care of my body.

- I nurture my body with sound habits.

- I deserve a clean, fit body.

- I can alter my habits by altering my mind.

- I respect and honor myself always.

- I'm solid enough to defeat any challenge.

- I trust in my might to do anything I wish.

How to use reinforcement

Affirmations work best when they're recited repeatedly and while giving your full focus to them. Not only should you say the words, all the same you ought to likewise do your best to bring forward the corresponding sense associated with the words. For example, if you state, "I feel so strong and empowered" you ought to in reality make an attempt to feel that way. This does take practice if you're not used to controlling your emotional state, all the same it gets easier the more you do it.

Constant repetition a lot of times a day is crucial also, because you're trying to reverse existing beliefs in your subconscious mind.

The illustration affirmations here will assist you in getting you started; all the same feel free to compose your own too!

Affirmations do take time to totally sink in to your subconscious mind, all the same just like your old notions were formed; consistent repetition and reinforcement will assist them in becoming lasting.

Chapter 6:

Healthy Habits For A Better Life

Synopsis

Do you sweat the small stuff? Do you find strain has increased in your life due to gloomy episodes? Are you searching for a fresh life-style, yet find it hard to relax and find answers?

We have many choices in the world, which gives us the convenience of having fun while choosing a better life-style. When altering your life-style you'll likely have to make decisions that will be hard, yet you are able to do it if you consider yourself and not others.

Remember stress leads to smoking.

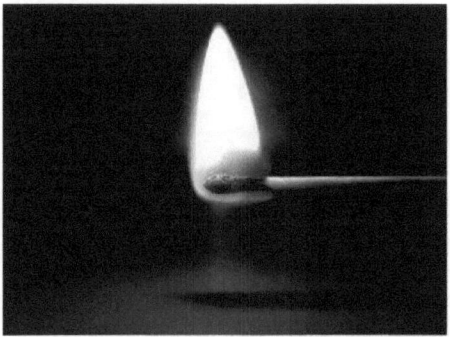

Change It

We all have to learn how to relax and take care of ourselves so we may see a brighter future.

We all have to make our life simple. Keeping it simple will help reduce stress. Occasionally we have to give up our homes. The stress of preserving, our home increases. Money commonly becomes a big issue, which causes stress. The care and taxes alone are very stressful for somebody that's living on little money these days.

How to choose:

Do you plan to stay in the same area you live now? Do you want to live in a better climate? The questions demand an answer before mortgaging your home. If you plan to move to a better climate to live healthier, think about the climate.

A lot of us suffer from allergies, hay fever, or other ailments due to climate changes. If you plan to live healthier and reduce, your risks of upper respiratory conditions then consider your options before making a choice to move. You need to consider your budget also. If you're living a fixed-income, consider the low-cost housing projects.

Don't get me wrong there will constantly be some stress in your life that you will not have control of. Now that you've made one of the biggest decision about where you going to live, begin thinking about enjoying life.

Join an exercise group or get a few neighbors to join you for a walk. Walk on sunny days so your body gets natural vitamin D from the sun-rays. The vitamins will help keep your bones strong. Exercising helps keep us fit and is a great way to meet new individuals while having fun.

Don't forget to watch your diet and make certain your getting enough vitamins to keep yourself healthy. If not sure what vitamins you need and how much consult your doctor he may help you make a plan or send you to a dietician to help you with it.

Occasionally we don't eat as much, especially if we have been a smoker so supplement vitamins are needed. Your family health professional can help you with this too.

The world is filled with assorted life-styles, so make your life your own by remaining healthy and avoid sweating the small stuff. Making sound decisions is a great beginning to living free, which promotes health.

Wrapping Up

Daily the ex-smoker should awaken thinking that he isn't going to smoke that day. And every night before he turns in he should to compliment himself for sticking to his goal. As pride is crucial in remaining free from cigarettes.

Not only is it essential, but it's well deserved. For anyone who's quit smoking has broken free from a really powerful addiction. For the first time in a long time, he's gained control over his life, rather than being commanded by his cigarette. For this, he should to be proud.

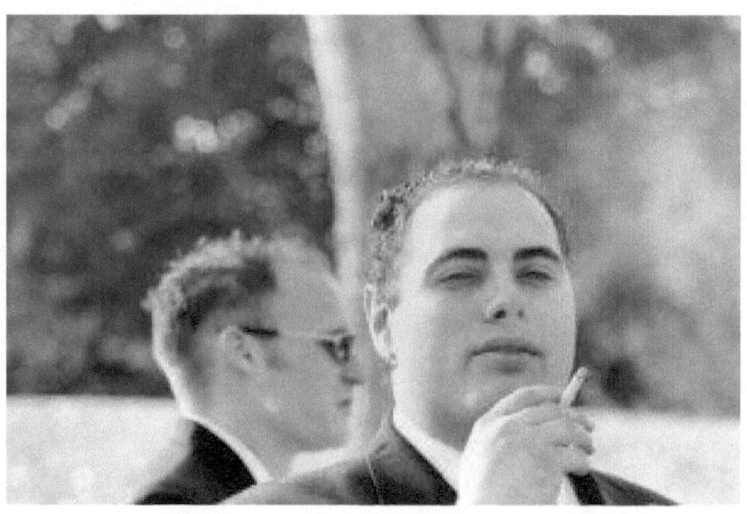